MIND DIET COOKBOOK FOR SENIORS AFTER 60

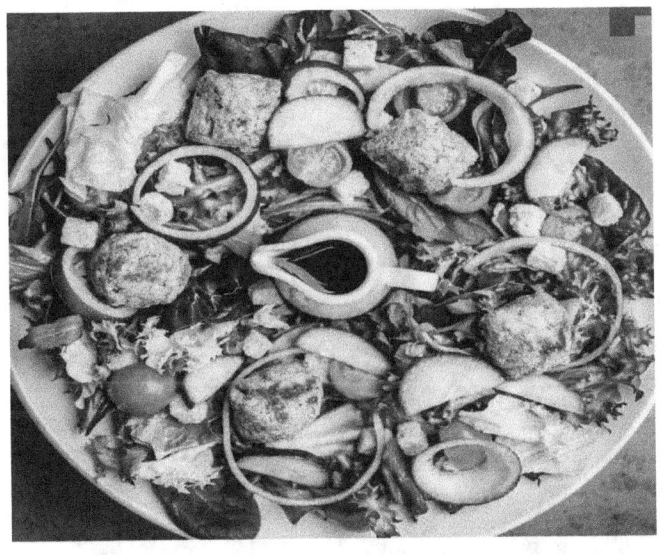

30 Quick and Delicious Brain Boosting Recipes with an easy guide to help fight memory disorders to improve brain function / with 7 weeks meal plan.

CARLY EVELYN

Disclaimer: The information provided in this cookbook is for educational purposes only and is not intended as a substitute for professional medical advice, diagnosis, or treatment

SCAN TO GET MORE BOOKS FROM THIS AUTHOR

IF YOU ARE STUCK, WHILE PREPARING ANY RECIPES IN THIS COOKBOOK, YOU CAN REACH THE AUTHOR AT CARLYEVLCUISINEGUIDE@GMAIL.COM FOR GUIDANCE

TABLE OF CONTENT

TABLE OF CONTENT

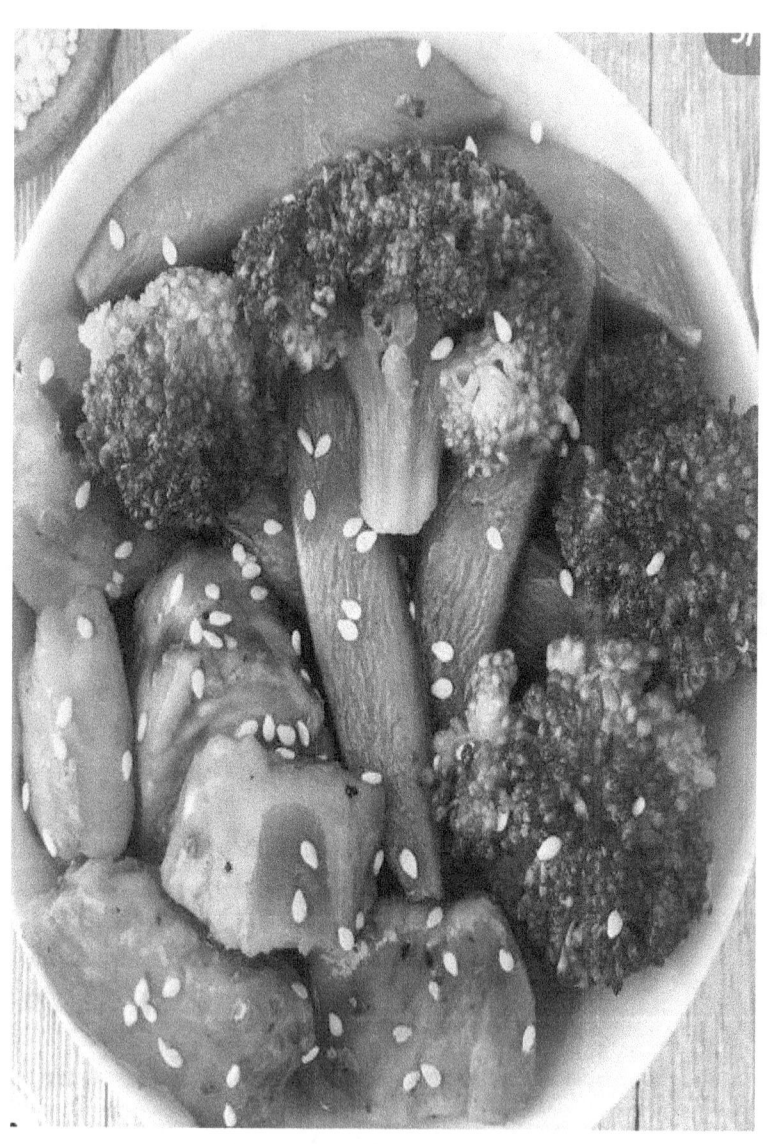

INTRODUCTION

Seniors often suffer from the silent adversary of mind disease, a shadow that dims the clarity of cherished memories and clouds the once-sharp minds of those who have lived a lifetime. In the heart of this struggle was an old man named Robert, whose vibrant past was slowly succumbing to the relentless grip of cognitive decline.

As the fog settled in, Robert's days became a maze of forgetfulness. Faces that once held stories became unfamiliar, and the threads of connection that wove through his life began to unravel. Determined not to surrender to this encroaching darkness, Robert sought solace in the promise of a brighter tomorrow.

Armed with a steadfast spirit and the guidance of a MIND diet cookbook, Robert embarked on a journey of transformation. The pages of the cookbook unfolded like a roadmap to rejuvenation, with recipes carefully crafted to nourish not only the body but the intricate workings of the mind.

Berries, leafy greens, and the omega-3 dance of fish became the allies in Robert's quest for mental clarity. Each meal, infused with the wisdom of the MIND diet, became a testament to his resilience. Slowly but surely, the fog that had settled over his mind began to lift.

The once-forgotten stories found their way back into Robert's consciousness, and the maze of uncertainty began to unravel. Faces, once elusive, became familiar once more. The town that had seemed distant in the haze became vivid and tangible.

Robert's journey was not just a personal triumph; it echoed through the community, a beacon of hope for others grappling with the same adversary. The whispers of mind disease that once haunted him were replaced by the hum of resilience and the transformative power of mindful nutrition.

In the quiet triumph of an old man's determination, a narrative unfolded—a story of reversal and management, where the right diet became a key to unlocking the doors of mental clarity. And so, against the backdrop of aging, Robert discovered that the chapters of the mind could be rewritten with each carefully chosen ingredient, offering a recipe not just for nourishment but for a rekindled vibrancy in the golden years.

GUIDE TO UNDERSTAND MIND DISEASE BETTER.

As you age, your cognitive health becomes increasingly important. One common concern is the Mind Diet Disease, a term encompassing various cognitive challenges experienced by you seniors over the age of 60. These challenges can range from mild cognitive impairment to more severe conditions like dementia and Alzheimer's.

Types of Mind Diet Disease: Navigating the Spectrum

Within the realm of Mind Diet Disease, there exists a spectrum of conditions. Mild cognitive impairment often serves as an early warning sign, indicating subtle changes in memory and thinking abilities. Progressing along the spectrum, which can make you encounter Alzheimer's disease, a form of dementia characterized by more profound cognitive decline, affecting daily life.

Causes of Mind Diet Disease: Unraveling the Complexity

Understanding the causes of Mind Diet Disease is crucial for prevention and intervention. While aging is a natural factor, genetic predispositions, lifestyle choices, and environmental factors also play significant roles. Unraveling the complexity of these causes can guide you in developing strategies to mitigate the risk and impact of Mind Diet Disease.

Symptoms: Recognizing the Early Signs

Early detection is key in managing Mind Diet Disease. Recognizing the symptoms allows for timely intervention and improved quality of life. Common signs include memory loss, confusion, changes in mood and behavior, and difficulty in performing familiar tasks. By staying informed about these indicators, you and your loved ones can take proactive steps toward maintaining cognitive health.

Preventive Measures: Nourishing the Mind

Fortunately, there are several preventive measures that can be incorporated into daily life to promote cognitive well-being. A fundamental aspect is adopting a Mind Diet, rich in brain-boosting nutrients. This diet emphasizes fruits, vegetables, whole grains, nuts, and fish—foods known for their positive impact on cognitive function. Regular physical exercise, mental stimulation, adequate sleep, and social engagement also contribute significantly to preventive measures.

Finally, understanding Mind Diet Disease involves exploring its types, delving into the causes, recognizing symptoms, and embracing preventive measures. By taking a holistic approach that addresses both lifestyle choices and dietary habits, these can empower seniors to age gracefully, preserving their cognitive abilities and enhancing their overall quality of life.

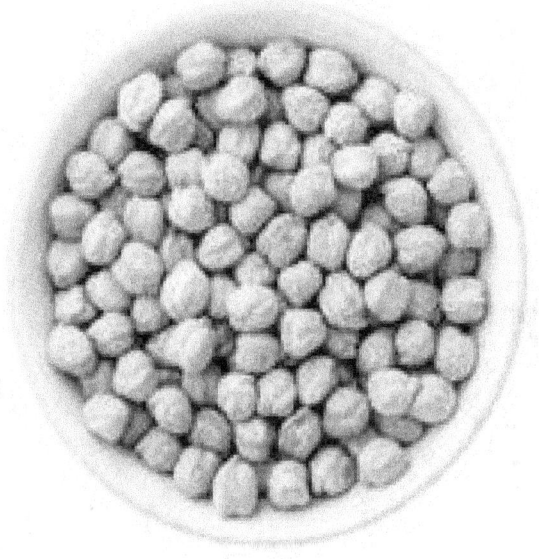

Chickpeas

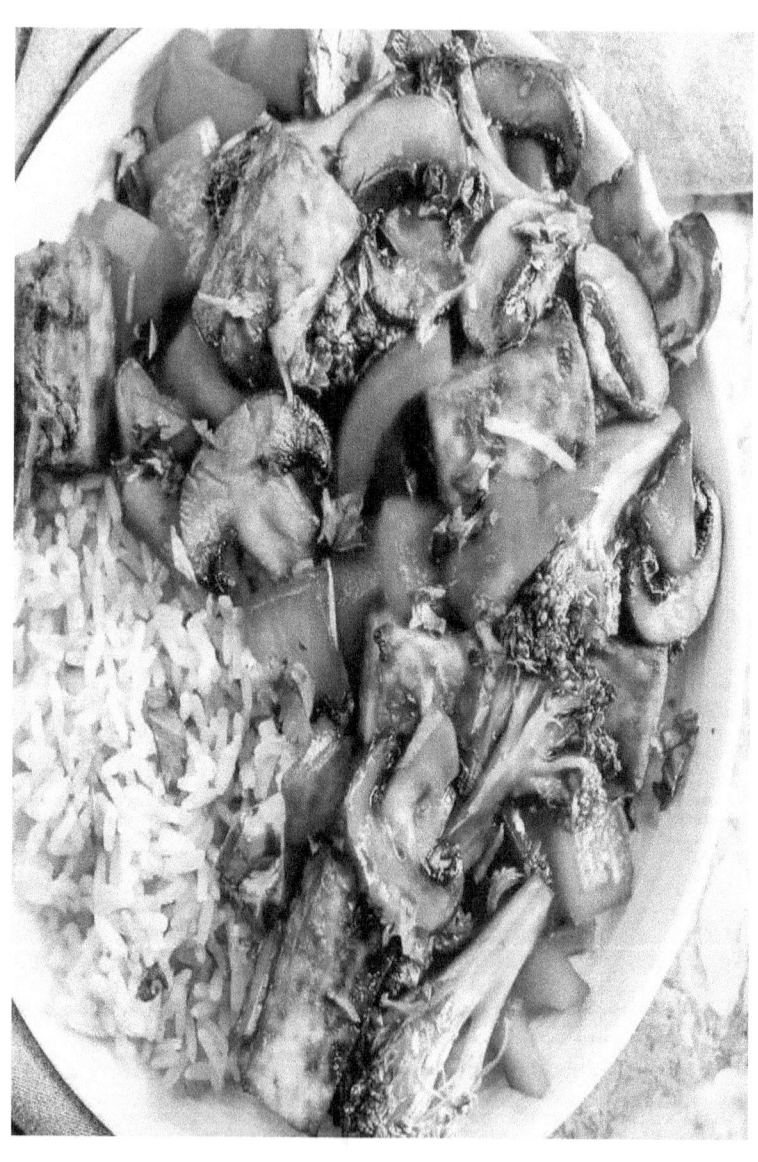

Chapter 1

CORE BENEFITS OF FOLLOWING A MIND DISEASE DIET

Adopting a mind disease diet for seniors can offer a range of core benefits that contribute to overall well-being and cognitive health. Here are some key advantages:

Brain Health Preservation:

A mind disease diet prioritizes foods rich in antioxidants, vitamins, and minerals known to support brain health. These nutrients help protect against oxidative stress, inflammation, and age-related damage, preserving cognitive function.

Reduced Risk of Cognitive Decline:

The inclusion of brain-boosting nutrients, such as omega-3 fatty acids and antioxidants, has been associated with a reduced risk of cognitive decline and disorders like Alzheimer's. The diet's emphasis on neuroprotective foods acts as a preventive measure against age-related cognitive challenges.

Improved Memory and Cognitive Performance:

The nutrient-dense nature of a mind disease diet provides essential building blocks for optimal brain function. Regular consumption of foods like berries and fatty fish has been linked to improved memory, concentration, and overall cognitive performance.

Enhanced Mood and Emotional Well-being:

Certain nutrients in the mind disease diet, such as omega-3 fatty acids and serotonin-boosting foods, have positive effects on mood regulation. Maintaining emotional well-being is crucial for seniors, contributing to a higher quality of life.

Heart Health Benefits:

Many components of a mind disease diet, including fruits, vegetables, and fatty fish, also promote heart health. A healthy cardiovascular system supports efficient blood flow to the brain, ensuring optimal oxygen and nutrient delivery for cognitive function.

Stabilized Blood Sugar Levels:

The emphasis on whole grains and balanced nutrition helps regulate blood sugar levels. Stable blood sugar is essential for preventing cognitive decline and maintaining energy levels throughout the day.

Weight Management:

Following a mind disease diet encourages a balanced and nutritious approach to eating, which can contribute to weight management. Maintaining a healthy weight is associated with a lower risk of various health issues, including cognitive decline.

Anti-Inflammatory Effects:

Chronic inflammation has been linked to various health problems, including cognitive decline. The anti-inflammatory properties of certain foods in the mind disease diet, such as turmeric and fatty fish, can help mitigate inflammation in the body and brain.

Improved Gut Health:
The inclusion of fiber-rich foods, such as fruits, vegetables, and whole grains, supports a healthy gut microbiome. Emerging research suggests a strong connection between gut health and brain function, highlighting the importance of a well-balanced diet.

Long-term Cognitive Resilience:
By adopting a mind disease diet, seniors invest in their long-term cognitive resilience. The cumulative effects of nutrient-rich foods and healthy lifestyle choices contribute to a robust defense against age-related cognitive challenges.

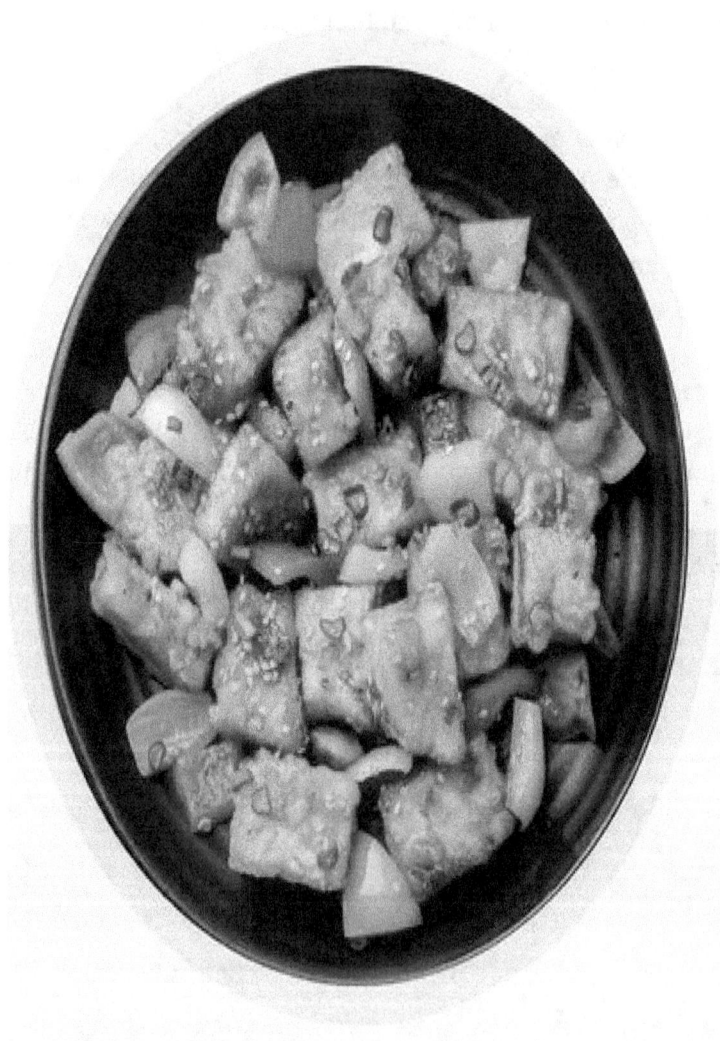

ACHIEVING OPTIMUM HEALTH WITH MIND DIET: FOODS TO EAT AND AVOID
Nourishing the Mind: A Guide to Optimum Cognitive Health

As you delve into the realm of a mind disease diet, it's essential to focus on foods that contribute to optimum cognitive health. Adopting a diet rich in brain-boosting nutrients can significantly impact your overall well-being. Here's a guide to the foods to embrace and those to avoid for a healthy mind:

FOODS TO EMBRACE:

Leafy Greens:
Leafy greens like spinach, kale, and Swiss chard are packed with antioxidants, vitamins, and minerals. These nutrients play a crucial role in supporting brain health and protecting against oxidative stress.

Berries:
Blueberries, strawberries, and blackberries are not only delicious but also potent allies for cognitive function. Rich in antioxidants, they have been linked to improved memory and delayed cognitive decline

Fatty Fish:
Salmon, trout, and sardines are abundant in omega-3 fatty acids, particularly DHA. These essential fats are

fundamental for maintaining the structure and function of brain cells, promoting communication between nerve cells.

Whole Grains:
Opt for whole grains like brown rice, quinoa, and oats. These grains provide a steady supply of energy to the brain and contain essential nutrients such as fiber, vitamins, and antioxidants.

Nuts and Seeds:
Almonds, walnuts, flaxseeds, and chia seeds are excellent sources of omega-3 fatty acids, antioxidants, and vitamin E. Incorporating a handful of these into your daily diet can contribute to improved cognitive performance.

Avocados:
Avocados are not only creamy and delicious but also rich in monounsaturated fats, which support healthy blood flow, crucial for optimal brain function.

Turmeric:
Curcumin, the active compound in turmeric, has anti-inflammatory and antioxidant benefits. Including turmeric in your diet may help protect the brain from inflammation and oxidative stress.

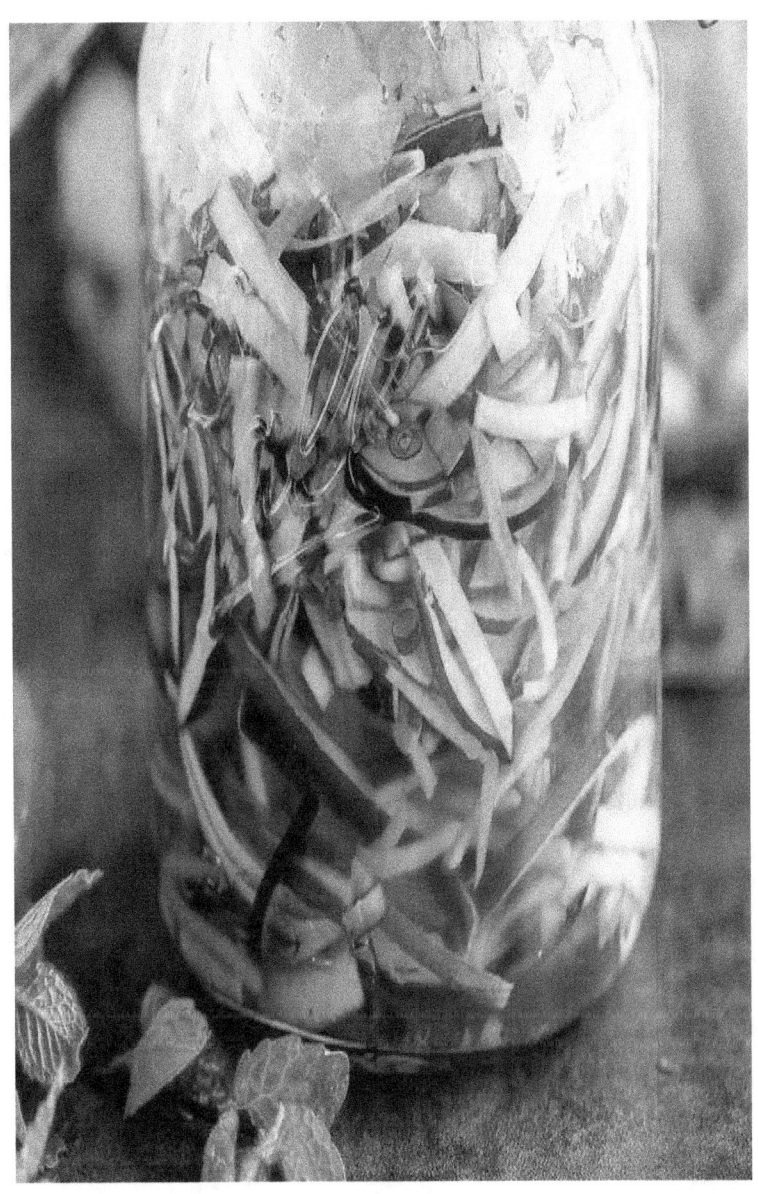

FOODS TO RESTRICT OR AVOID:

Processed Foods:
Highly processed foods often contain additives, preservatives, and unhealthy fats that may contribute to inflammation and negatively impact cognitive health. Minimize the consumption of packaged snacks and convenience foods.

Sugary Treats:
Excessive sugar intake has been linked to cognitive decline. Reduce the consumption of sugary beverages, candies, and desserts, opting for natural sweeteners like honey or maple syrup in moderation.

Red and Processed Meat:
High intake of red and processed meats has been associated with an increased risk of cognitive decline. Consider leaner protein sources such as poultry, fish, and plant-based alternatives.

Trans Fats:
Found in some margarines and commercially baked goods, trans fats can have detrimental effects on cognitive function. Check labels and opt for healthier fats like those found in olive oil or avocados.

Excessive Alcohol:
While moderate alcohol consumption may have some health benefits, excessive intake can impair cognitive function. It's advisable to limit alcohol consumption to support overall brain health.

In short, a mind disease diet is centered around nourishing the mind with nutrient-dense foods that support cognitive function and protect against age-related decline. By incorporating these wholesome choices into your daily meals and being mindful of foods to limit or avoid, you can take proactive steps toward achieving optimum cognitive health.

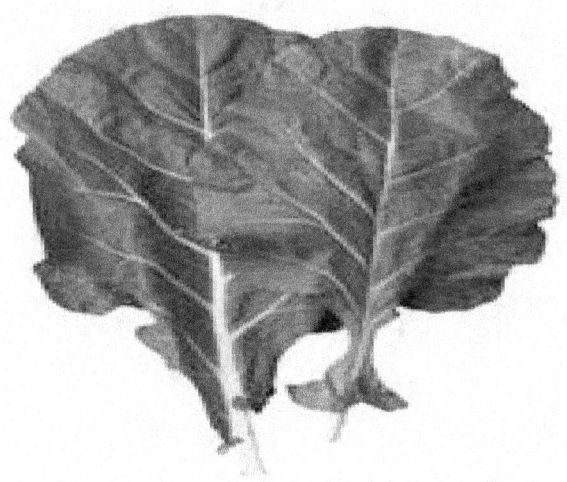

Collard Greens

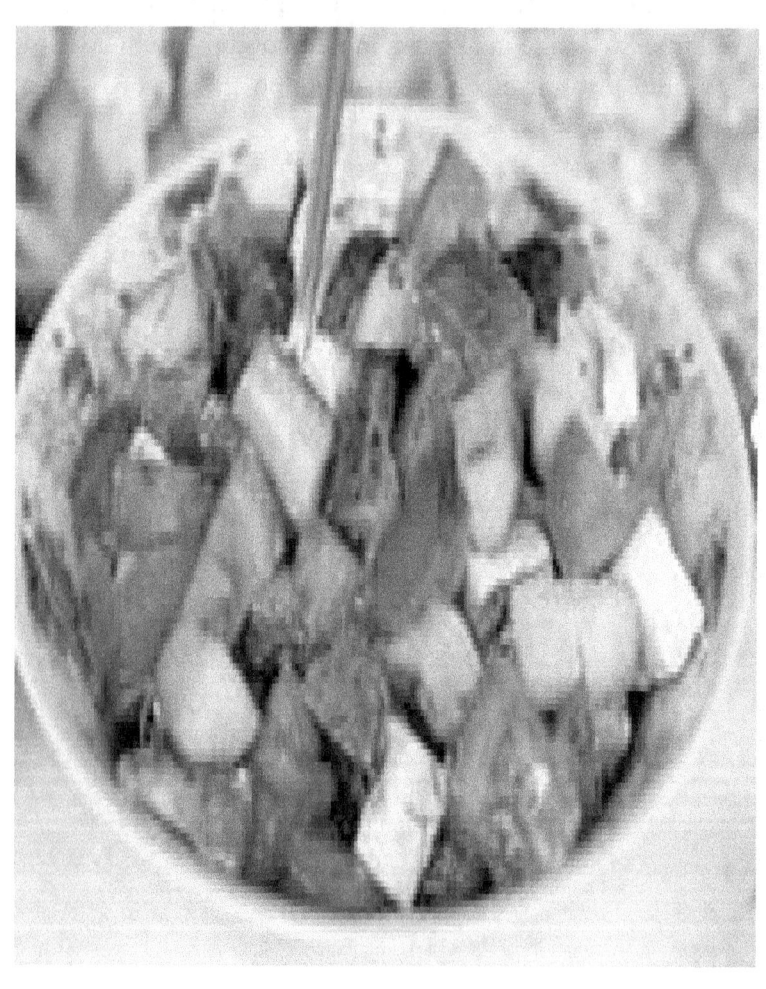

Chapter 2

20 HEALTHY SHOPPING INGREDIENTS OR LISTS FOR MIND DISEASE DIET

Here's a list of 20 healthy ingredients for a mind disease diet to include in your shopping list:

Fatty Fish:
Salmon
Trout
Sardines
These are rich in omega-3 fatty acids, essential for brain health.

Berries:
Blueberries
Strawberries
Blackberries
Packed with antioxidants, berries are known to support cognitive function.

Leafy Greens:
Spinach
Kale
Swiss Chard
Leafy greens are abundant in vitamins, minerals, and antioxidants crucial for brain health.

Whole Grains:

Brown rice
Quinoa
Oats
Whole grains provide a steady supply of energy and essential nutrients for optimal brain function.

Nuts and Seeds:
Almonds
Walnuts
Flaxseeds
Chia Seeds
These are excellent sources of healthy fats, antioxidants, and essential nutrients for brain health.

Avocados:
Rich in monounsaturated fats, avocados support healthy blood flow to the brain.

Turmeric:
Ground turmeric
Fresh turmeric
The active compound curcumin in turmeric has anti-inflammatory and antioxidant properties.

Broccoli:
High in antioxidants and vitamin K, broccoli is a nutritious addition to support overall health.

Poultry:
Chicken
Turkey
Lean protein sources like poultry provide essential amino acids for neurotransmitter synthesis.

Beans and Legumes:
Chickpeas
Lentils
Black beans
Beans and legumes are rich in fiber and protein, supporting overall health.

Tomatoes:
Rich in antioxidants, especially lycopene, tomatoes contribute to brain health.

Dark Chocolate (in moderation):
Dark chocolate contains flavonoids that may have cognitive benefits. Choose varieties with higher cocoa content.

Eggs:
Eggs are a good source of choline, a nutrient important for brain health.

Olive Oil:
Extra virgin olive oil is rich in monounsaturated fats and has anti-inflammatory properties.

Green Tea:
Green tea contains antioxidants and a small amount of caffeine, promoting alertness and cognitive function.

Low-Fat Dairy:
Greek yogurt
Low-fat milk
These provide calcium and vitamin D, essential for overall health.

Colorful Vegetables:
Bell peppers
Carrots
Beets
Include a variety of colorful vegetables for a range of antioxidants and nutrients.

Lean Red Meat (in moderation):
Opt for lean cuts of red meat for a source of iron and zinc, important for cognitive health.

Oranges and Citrus Fruits:
High in vitamin C, citrus fruits contribute to overall immune health.

Water:
While not a traditional ingredient, staying hydrated is crucial for cognitive function and overall well-being.

Chapter 3

*SERIAL 7 DAY SAMPLE MIND DISEASE
DIET MEAL PLAN.*

Here's a 7-day sample mind disease diet meal plan for breakfast, lunch, and dinner:

Day 1
Breakfast:
Greek Yogurt Parfait with Berries and Almonds
Lunch:
Grilled Salmon Salad with Leafy Greens, Cherry Tomatoes, and Avocado
Dinner:
Quinoa-Stuffed Bell Peppers with Lean Ground Turkey and Black Beans

Day 2
Breakfast:
Oatmeal with Chia Seeds, Walnuts, and Sliced Banana
Lunch:
Chickpea and Spinach Curry with Brown Rice
Dinner:
Baked Cod with Roasted Vegetables (Broccoli, Carrots, and Bell Peppers)

Day 3
Breakfast:
Smoothie with Spinach, Blueberries, Greek Yogurt, and Flaxseeds

Lunch:
Lentil Soup with Whole Grain Crackers
Dinner:
Grilled Chicken Breast with Quinoa and Steamed Asparagus

Day 4
Breakfast:
Whole Grain Toast with Smashed Avocado and Poached Eggs
Lunch:
Turkey and Vegetable Wrap with Whole Wheat Tortilla
Dinner:
Stir-Fried Tofu with Mixed Vegetables and Brown Ric

Day 5
Breakfast:
Berry and Spinach Smoothie Bowl with Almond Butter Drizzle
Lunch:
Quinoa Salad with Cherry Tomatoes, Cucumber, Feta, and Olive Oil Dressing
Dinner:
Baked Chicken Thighs with Sweet Potato Wedges and Green Beans

Day 6
Breakfast:
Whole Grain Pancakes with Fresh Berries and a Dollop of Greek Yogurt

Lunch:
Shrimp and Vegetable Stir-Fry with Quinoa
Dinner:
Grilled Swordfish with Mango Salsa and Steamed Broccoli

Day 7
Breakfast:
Scrambled Eggs with Spinach and Tomatoes, served with Whole Grain Toast
Lunch:
Chickpea Salad with Avocado, Cherry Tomatoes, and Lime Dressing
Dinner:
Vegetable and Tofu Curry with Brown Rice

Feel free to adjust portion sizes based on your needs and preferences. Additionally, incorporate snacks like nuts, fresh fruits, or yogurt throughout the day for added nutrition and energy.

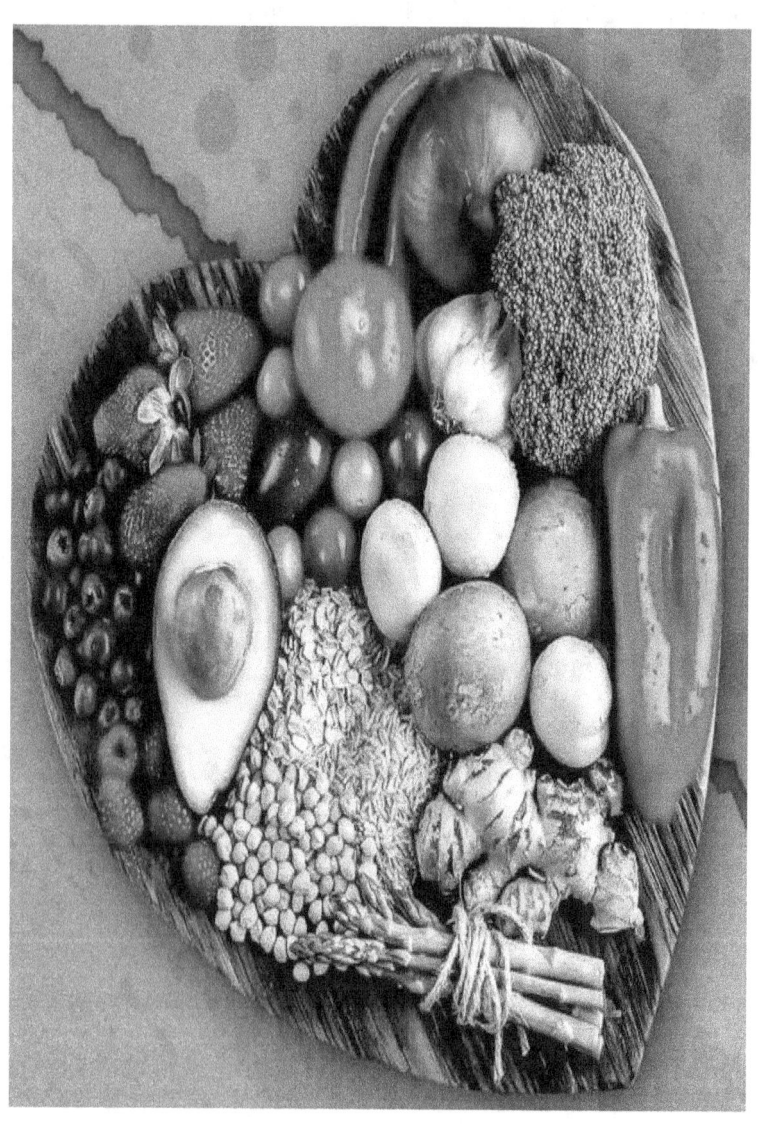

Chapter 4

MIND DIET BREAKFAST RECIPES

1. Greek Yogurt Parfait with Berries and Almonds

Ingredients:

1 cup Greek yogurt

1/2 cup mixed berries (blueberries, strawberries, blackberries)

1/4 cup almonds, sliced

1 tablespoon honey

Preparation:

In a glass or bowl, layer half of the Greek yogurt.

Add half of the mixed berries on top of the yogurt.

Sprinkle half of the sliced almonds.

Drizzle with half of the honey.

Repeat the layers with the remaining ingredients.

Serve immediately.

Nutritional Value (per serving):

Calories: 350

Protein: 20g

Fiber: 6g

Healthy Fats: 15g

Calcium: 25% DV

Serving Measurements: 1 serving

Cooking Time: 5 minutes

2. Oatmeal with Chia Seeds, Walnuts, and Sliced Banana

Ingredients:

1/2 cup rolled oats

1 cup milk (dairy or plant-based)

1 tablespoon chia seeds

1/4 cup walnuts, chopped

1 medium banana, sliced

Preparation:

In a saucepan, combine rolled oats and milk.

Cook over medium heat, stirring frequently until the oats are cooked and the mixture thickens.

Remove from heat and stir in chia seeds.

Transfer to a bowl and top with chopped walnuts and sliced banana.

Nutritional Value (per serving):

Calories: 400

Protein: 12g

Fiber: 9g

Healthy Fats: 15g

Potassium: 15% DV

Serving Measurements: 1 serving

Cooking Time: 10 minutes

3. Smoothie with Spinach, Blueberries, Greek Yogurt, and Flaxseeds

Ingredients:

1 cup spinach

1/2 cup blueberries

1/2 cup Greek yogurt

1 tablespoon flaxseeds

1 cup water or almond milk

Preparation:

In a blender, combine spinach, blueberries, Greek yogurt, flaxseeds, and water or almond milk.

Blend until smooth and creamy.

Pour into a glass and serve immediately.

Nutritional Value (per serving):

Calories: 250

Protein: 15g

Fiber: 8g

Healthy Fats: 10g

Vitamin C: 30% DV

Serving Measurements: 1 serving

Cooking Time: 5 minutes

4. Whole Grain Pancakes with Fresh Berries and Greek Yogurt

Ingredients:

1 cup whole wheat flour

1 tablespoon baking powder

1 tablespoon honey

1 cup milk (dairy or plant-based)

1 egg

Fresh berries for topping

Greek yogurt for topping

Preparation:

In a bowl, whisk together whole wheat flour, baking powder, honey, milk, and egg until well combined.

Heat a griddle or non-stick pan over medium heat.

Pour 1/4 cup of batter onto the griddle for each pancake.

Cook until bubbles form on the surface, then flip and cook the other side.

Serve pancakes topped with fresh berries and a dollop of Greek yogurt.

Nutritional Value (per serving):

Calories: 300

Protein: 12g

Fiber: 6g

Healthy Fats: 8g

Iron: 15% DV

Serving Measurements: 2-3 pancakes per serving

Cooking Time: 15 minutes

5. Scrambled Eggs with Spinach and Tomatoes, served with Whole Grain Toast

Ingredients:

2 large eggs

1 cup fresh spinach, chopped

1/2 cup cherry tomatoes, halved

1 tablespoon olive oil

Salt and pepper to taste

2 slices whole grain bread

Preparation:

In a pan, heat olive oil over medium heat.

Add spinach and tomatoes, sauté until spinach wilts and tomatoes soften.

In a bowl, beat eggs, season with salt and pepper, and pour over the veggies.

Scramble the eggs until cooked to your liking.

Toast whole grain bread slices and serve with scrambled eggs.

Nutritional Value (per serving):

Calories: 320

Protein: 15g

Fiber: 6g

Healthy Fats: 10g

Vitamin A: 50% DV

Serving Measurements: 1 serving

Cooking Time: 10 minutes

6. Chickpea and Spinach Curry with Brown Rice

Ingredients:

1 cup chickpeas (canned or cooked)

1 cup fresh spinach, chopped

1/2 cup diced tomatoes

1/4 cup diced onions

1 tablespoon curry powder

1 cup cooked brown rice

Preparation:

In a pan, sauté onions until translucent.

Add chickpeas, diced tomatoes, and curry powder. Cook until tomatoes break down.

Stir in chopped spinach and cook until wilted.

Serve over cooked brown rice.

Nutritional Value (per serving):

Calories: 380

Protein: 15g

Fiber: 12g

Healthy Fats: 8g

Iron: 20% DV

Serving Measurements: 1 serving

Cooking Time: 15 minutes

7. Whole Grain Toast with Smashed Avocado and Poached Eggs

Ingredients:

2 slices whole grain bread

1 ripe avocado

2 large eggs
Salt and pepper to taste
Optional toppings: red pepper flakes, cherry tomatoes
Preparation:
Toast whole grain bread slices.
While the bread is toasting, smash the ripe avocado and spread it over the toasted slices.
Poach the eggs to your liking and place them on top of the smashed avocado.
Season with salt and pepper and add optional toppings if desired.
Nutritional Value (per serving):
Calories: 400
Protein: 16g
Fiber: 10g
Healthy Fats: 20g
Vitamin E: 15% DV
Serving Measurements: 1 serving
Cooking Time: 10 minutes

8. Baked Chicken Thighs with Sweet Potato Wedges and Green Beans
Ingredients:
2 bone-in, skin-on chicken thighs
1 large sweet potato, cut into wedges
1 cup green beans, trimmed
1 tablespoon olive oil
Salt, pepper, garlic powder, and paprika to taste
Preparation:
Preheat oven to 400°F (200°C).
Season chicken thighs with salt, pepper, garlic powder, and paprika.
Toss sweet potato wedges and green beans with olive oil, salt, and pepper.
Place chicken thighs on a baking sheet and surround them with sweet potato wedges and green beans.
Bake for 30-35 minutes or until chicken is cooked through and vegetables are tender.
Nutritional Value (per serving):

Calories: 450
Protein: 25g
Fiber: 8g
Healthy Fats: 15g
Vitamin A: 200% DV
Serving Measurements: 1 serving
Cooking Time: 35 minutes

9. Chia Seed Pudding with Mixed Berries and Almond Butter

Ingredients:

3 tablespoons chia seeds

1 cup almond milk

1/2 teaspoon vanilla extract

1 tablespoon maple syrup

Mixed berries (strawberries, blueberries, raspberries)

1 tablespoon almond butter

Preparation:

In a bowl, mix chia seeds, almond milk, vanilla extract, and maple syrup.

Stir well and refrigerate overnight or for at least 4 hours until it thickens.

In the morning, layer the chia seed pudding with mixed berries and top with a dollop of almond butter.

Nutritional Value (per serving):

Calories: 280

Protein: 8g

Fiber: 14g

Healthy Fats: 12g

Calcium: 30% DV

Serving Measurements: 1 serving

Cooking Time: 5 minutes (plus overnight refrigeration)

10. Whole Grain Breakfast Burrito with Eggs and Black Beans

Ingredients:

2 large eggs, scrambled

1/2 cup black beans, drained and rinsed

1/4 cup diced tomatoes

1/4 cup diced bell peppers

Whole wheat tortilla

Avocado slices for topping

Fresh cilantro for garnish

Preparation:

In a pan, scramble the eggs until cooked through.

Heat black beans, diced tomatoes, and bell peppers in the same pan.

Warm the whole wheat tortilla and assemble the burrito with scrambled eggs, black bean mixture, avocado slices, and fresh cilantro.

Nutritional Value (per serving):

Calories: 380

Protein: 18g

Fiber: 12g

Healthy Fats: 15g

Vitamin C: 40% DV

Serving Measurements: 1 serving

Cooking Time: 10 minutes

MIND DIET LUNCH RECIPES
1. Grilled Salmon Salad with Avocado and Quinoa
Ingredients:
1 salmon fillet (6 oz)
1 cup cooked quinoa
2 cups mixed salad greens
1/2 avocado, sliced
1/4 cup cherry tomatoes, halved
1 tablespoon olive oil
1 tablespoon lemon juice
Salt and pepper to taste
Preparation
Season the salmon fillet with salt and pepper.
Grill the salmon for 3-4 minutes per side until cooked.
In a bowl, combine quinoa, salad greens, avocado, and cherry tomatoes.
Place the grilled salmon on top.
Drizzle with olive oil and lemon juice.
Toss gently and serve.
Nutritional Value (per serving):
Calories: 500
Protein: 30g
Fiber: 8g
Healthy Fats: 25g
Omega-3 Fatty Acids: 1.5g
Serving Measurements: 1 serving
Cooking Time: 10 minutes

2. Chickpea and Spinach Quinoa Bowl

Ingredients:

1 cup cooked quinoa

1 cup chickpeas (canned, drained, and rinsed)

2 cups fresh spinach

1/2 cup diced cucumber

1/4 cup feta cheese, crumbled

1 tablespoon olive oil

1 tablespoon balsamic vinegar

Salt and pepper to taste

Preparation:

In a bowl, combine quinoa, chickpeas, fresh spinach, cucumber, and feta cheese.

Drizzle with olive oil and balsamic vinegar.

Season with salt and pepper.

Toss gently and serve.

Nutritional Value (per serving):

Calories: 450

Protein: 18g

Fiber: 12g

Healthy Fats: 15g

Iron: 2.5mg

Serving Measurements: 1 serving

Cooking Time: 15 minutes

3. Turkey and Vegetable Wrap with Whole Wheat Tortilla

Ingredients:

4 oz lean ground turkey

1 whole wheat tortilla

1/2 cup mixed bell peppers, thinly sliced

1/4 cup red onion, thinly sliced

1/4 cup hummus

1 tablespoon olive oil

1 teaspoon taco seasoning

Preparation:

In a skillet, cook ground turkey with olive oil and taco seasoning until browned.

Warm the whole wheat tortilla.

Spread hummus on the tortilla.

Layer the cooked turkey, mixed bell peppers, and red onion.

Roll up the tortilla to form a wrap.

Nutritional Value (per serving):

Calories: 380

Protein: 25g

Fiber: 8g

Healthy Fats: 18g

Vitamin C: 40% DV

Serving Measurements: 1 serving

Cooking Time: 15 minutes

4. Mediterranean Quinoa Salad with Chicken

Ingredients:

1 cup cooked quinoa

4 oz grilled chicken breast, sliced

1/2 cup cherry tomatoes, halved

1/4 cup cucumber, diced

1/4 cup Kalamata olives, sliced

2 tablespoons feta cheese, crumbled

1 tablespoon olive oil

1 tablespoon red wine vinegar

Fresh oregano for garnish

Salt and pepper to taste

Preparation:

In a bowl, combine quinoa, grilled chicken, cherry tomatoes, cucumber, olives, and feta cheese.

Drizzle with olive oil and red wine vinegar.

Season with salt and pepper.

Toss gently and garnish with fresh oregano.

Nutritional Value (per serving):

Calories: 420

Protein: 30g

Fiber: 8g

Healthy Fats: 18g

Calcium: 15% DV

Serving Measurements: 1 serving

Cooking Time: 20 minutes

5. Vegetarian Stir-Fried Tofu with Brown Rice

Ingredients:
1 cup extra-firm tofu, cubed
1 cup broccoli florets
1/2 cup sliced bell peppers (assorted colors)
1/4 cup carrots, julienned
2 tablespoons soy sauce
1 tablespoon sesame oil
1 tablespoon rice vinegar
1 teaspoon ginger, minced
1 teaspoon garlic, minced
1 cup cooked brown rice

Preparation:
In a pan, sauté tofu cubes until golden brown.
Add broccoli, bell peppers, and carrots to the pan.
In a small bowl, mix soy sauce, sesame oil, rice vinegar, ginger, and garlic.
Pour the sauce over the tofu and vegetables, stir-frying until everything is well-coated.
Serve over cooked brown rice.

Nutritional Value (per serving):
Calories: 420
Protein: 20g
Fiber: 10g
Healthy Fats: 15g
Iron: 3.5mg
Serving Measurements: 1 serving
Cooking Time: 15 minutes

6. Mango and Avocado Quinoa Salad with Shrimp

Ingredients:

4 oz shrimp, peeled and deveined

1 cup cooked quinoa

1/2 cup mango, diced

1/2 avocado, sliced

1/4 cup red onion, finely chopped

1/4 cup cilantro, chopped

1 tablespoon olive oil

1 tablespoon lime juice

Salt and pepper to taste

Preparation:

Grill or sauté shrimp until cooked.

In a bowl, combine quinoa, mango, avocado, red onion, and cilantro.

Drizzle with olive oil and lime juice.

Season with salt and pepper.

Top the salad with cooked shrimp.

Nutritional Value (per serving):

Calories: 380

Protein: 25g

Fiber: 8g

Healthy Fats: 15g

Vitamin C: 30% DV

Serving Measurements: 1 serving

Cooking Time: 10 minutes

7. Whole Grain Wrap with Grilled Chicken and Hummus

Ingredients:

4 oz grilled chicken breast, sliced

1 whole grain wrap

1/4 cup hummus

1/2 cup mixed salad greens

1/4 cup cucumber, sliced

1/4 cup cherry tomatoes, halved

Preparation:

Warm the whole grain wrap.

Spread hummus on the wrap.

Layer grilled chicken, mixed salad greens, cucumber, and cherry tomatoes.

Roll up the wrap and slice in half.

Nutritional Value (per serving):

Calories: 380

Protein: 30g

Fiber: 8g

Healthy Fats: 15g

Vitamin A: 40% DV

Serving Measurements: 1 serving

Cooking Time: 15 minutes

8. Egg and Vegetable Quiche with Sweet Potato Crust

Ingredients:

4 large eggs

1 sweet potato, thinly sliced

1 cup broccoli florets

1/2 cup bell peppers, diced

1/4 cup feta cheese, crumbled

1 tablespoon olive oil

Salt and pepper to taste

Preparation:

Preheat oven to 375°F (190°C).

Layer thinly sliced sweet potato in a pie dish to form a crust.

In a skillet, sauté broccoli and bell peppers with olive oil until slightly softened.

Whisk eggs and season with salt and pepper.

Pour the egg mixture over the sweet potato crust.

Add sautéed vegetables and sprinkle with feta cheese.

Bake for 25-30 minutes or until the eggs are set.

Nutritional Value (per serving):

Calories: 350

Protein: 20g

Fiber: 6g

Healthy Fats: 15g

Vitamin C: 80% DV

Serving Measurements: 1 serving

Cooking Time: 35 minutes

9. Salmon and Quinoa Bowl with Roasted Vegetables:

Ingredients:

1 salmon fillet (6 oz)

1/2 cup cooked quinoa

1 cup mixed vegetables (zucchini, bell peppers, cherry tomatoes)

1 tablespoon olive oil

1 teaspoon dried herbs (such as thyme or rosemary)

Salt and pepper to taste

Preparation:

Preheat the oven to 400°F (200°C).

Place the salmon fillet and mixed vegetables on a baking sheet.

Drizzle with olive oil, sprinkle with dried herbs, salt, and pepper.

Roast in the oven for 15-20 minutes or until the salmon is cooked through.

Serve the roasted vegetables and salmon over cooked quinoa.

Nutritional Value (per serving):

Calories: 450

Protein: 30g

Fiber: 8g

Healthy Fats: 20g

Omega-3 Fatty Acids: 1.5g

Serving Measurements: 1 serving

Cooking Time: 20 minutes

10. Turkey and Quinoa Stuffed Bell Peppers
Ingredients:
1/2 cup quinoa, cooked
8 oz lean ground turkey
4 bell peppers, halved and seeds removed
1 cup black beans (canned, drained, and rinsed)
1/2 cup corn kernels (fresh or frozen)
1 cup tomato sauce
1 teaspoon cumin
1 teaspoon chili powder
Salt and pepper to taste
1/2 cup shredded cheddar cheese (optional)
Preparation:
Preheat the oven to 375°F (190°C).
In a skillet, cook ground turkey until browned.
Add cooked quinoa, black beans, corn, tomato sauce, cumin, chili powder, salt, and pepper to the skillet. Mix well.
Stuff each bell pepper half with the turkey and quinoa mixture.
Place the stuffed peppers in a baking dish and cover with foil.
Bake for 25-30 minutes. If desired, sprinkle shredded cheddar cheese on top during the last 5 minutes of baking until melted.
Serve hot.
Nutritional Value (per serving):
Calories: 380
Protein: 25g
Fiber: 10g

Healthy Fats: 12g
Vitamin A: 120% DV
Serving Measurements: 1 serving (2 stuffed pepper halves)
Cooking Time: 30 minutes

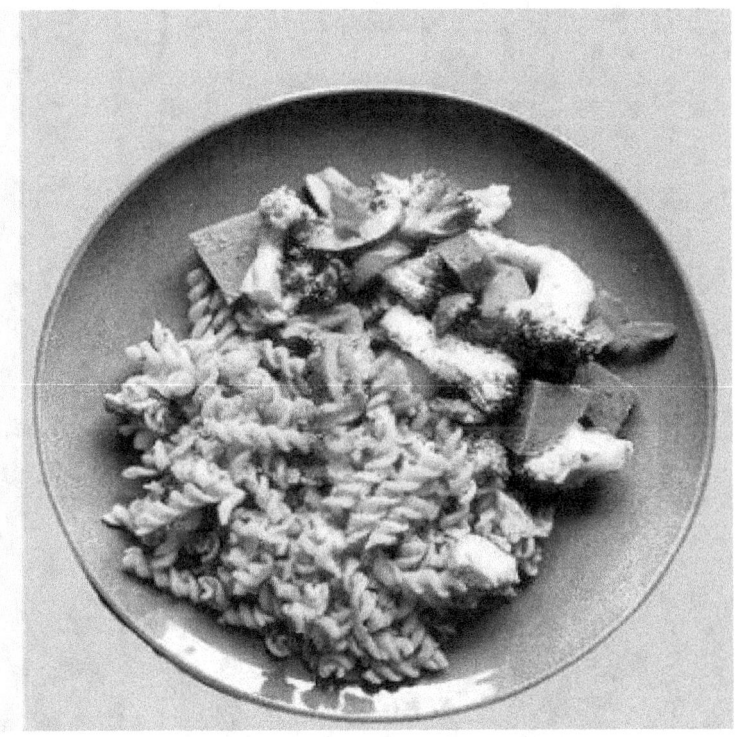

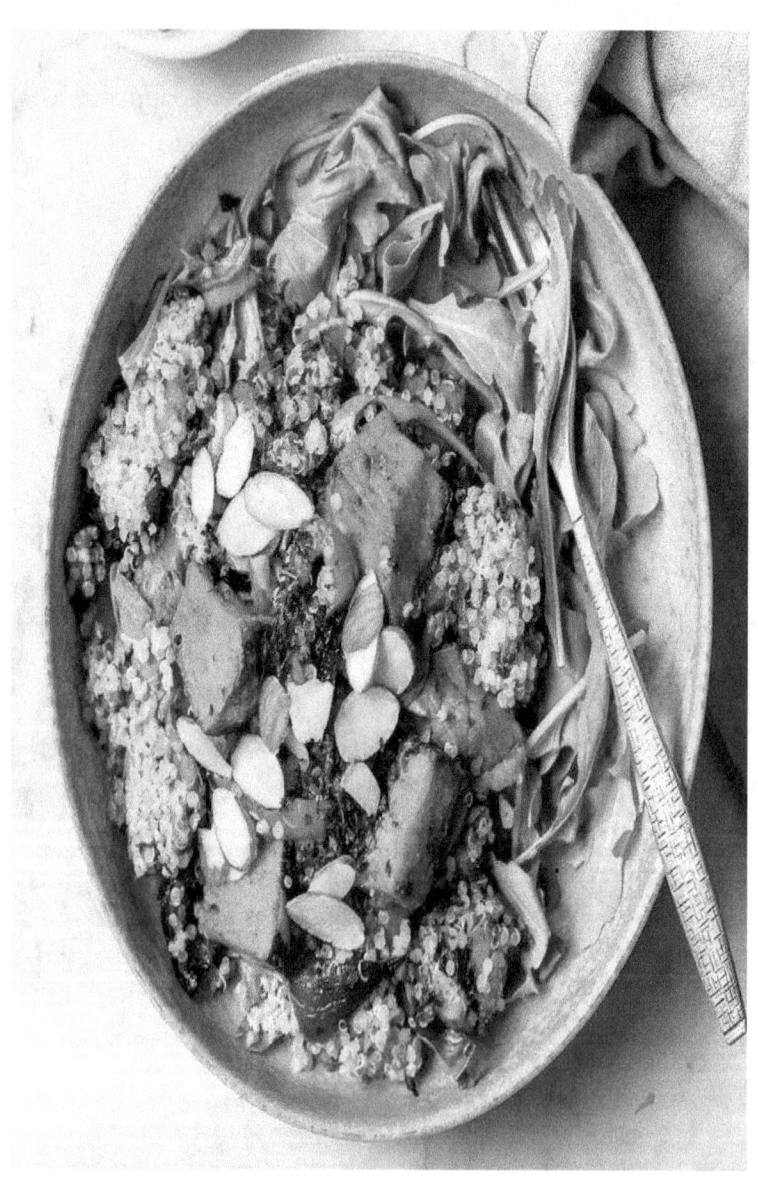

MIND DIET DINNER RECIPES

1. Salmon and Blueberry Salad

Ingredients:

2 salmon fillets (6 oz each)

2 cups mixed greens

1 cup fresh blueberries

1/4 cup chopped walnuts

1 tablespoon olive oil

1 tablespoon balsamic vinegar

Salt and pepper to taste

Preparation:

Preheat the oven to 375°F.

Season salmon fillets with salt and pepper, then bake for 15-18 minutes or until cooked through.

In a large bowl, toss mixed greens, blueberries, and chopped walnuts.

Flake the cooked salmon over the salad.

Drizzle olive oil and balsamic vinegar over the salad. Toss gently.

Serve immediately.

Nutritional Value:

Rich in omega-3 fatty acids, antioxidants, and vitamins.

Provides a good balance of healthy fats and proteins.

Serving:

Serves 2

Cooking Time:

20 minutes

2. Quinoa-Stuffed Bell Peppers

Ingredients:

1 cup quinoa
2 cups vegetable broth
4 bell peppers (any color)
1 can (15 oz) black beans, drained and rinsed
1 cup diced tomatoes
1 cup corn kernels
1 teaspoon cumin
1 teaspoon paprika
Salt and pepper to taste
1/2 cup shredded low-fat cheese (optional)

Preparation:

Preheat the oven to 400°F.

Cook quinoa in vegetable broth according to package instructions.

Cut the tops off bell peppers and remove seeds.

In a bowl, mix cooked quinoa, black beans, diced tomatoes, corn, cumin, paprika, salt, and pepper.

Stuff each bell pepper with the quinoa mixture.

Optional: Sprinkle shredded cheese on top.

Bake for 25-30 minutes or until peppers are tender.

Nutritional Value:

High in fiber, protein, and essential nutrients.

Low in saturated fats.

Serving:

Serves 4

Cooking Time:

40 minutes

3. Chicken and Vegetable Stir-Fry

Ingredients:

1 lb boneless, skinless chicken breast, thinly sliced

2 cups broccoli florets

1 red bell pepper, sliced

1 cup snap peas, trimmed

2 tablespoons low-sodium soy sauce

1 tablespoon olive oil

2 cloves garlic, minced

1 teaspoon ginger, grated

1 tablespoon sesame seeds (optional)

Brown rice or quinoa for serving

Preparation:

Heat olive oil in a wok or large skillet over medium-high heat.

Add sliced chicken and cook until browned and cooked through.

Add broccoli, bell pepper, snap peas, garlic, and ginger. Stir-fry for 5-7 minutes until vegetables are tender-crisp.

Drizzle soy sauce over the stir-fry and toss to combine.

Optional: Sprinkle sesame seeds on top.

Serve over brown rice or quinoa.

Nutritional Value:

High in lean protein, fiber, and essential vitamins.

Low in saturated fats.

Serving:

Serves 4

Cooking Time:

25 minutes

4. Sweet Potato and Spinach Frittata
Ingredients:
4 large eggs
1 cup sweet potatoes, diced and cooked
2 cups fresh spinach, chopped
1/2 cup feta cheese, crumbled
1/2 cup cherry tomatoes, halved
1 tablespoon olive oil
1 teaspoon dried thyme
Salt and pepper to taste
Preparation:
Preheat the oven to 350°F.
In an oven-safe skillet, heat olive oil over medium heat.
Add sweet potatoes, spinach, and cherry tomatoes. Cook until spinach wilts.
In a bowl, whisk eggs, thyme, salt, and pepper.
Pour the egg mixture over the vegetables in the skillet.
Sprinkle feta cheese on top.
Bake in the oven for 15-20 minutes or until the frittata is set.
Nutritional Value:
High in vitamins A, C, and iron.
Provides a good balance of protein and healthy fats.
Serving:
Serves 3-4
Cooking Time:
30 minutes

5. Baked Cod with Lemon and Herb Quinoa
Ingredients:
4 cod fillets (6 oz each)
1 cup quinoa
2 cups vegetable broth
1 lemon (zested and juiced)
2 tablespoons fresh parsley, chopped
1 tablespoon olive oil
2 cloves garlic, minced
Salt and pepper to taste
Preparation:
Preheat the oven to 400°F.
Season cod fillets with salt, pepper, and a drizzle of olive oil.
Place cod fillets on a baking sheet and bake for 15-18 minutes or until the fish flakes easily.
Cook quinoa in vegetable broth according to package instructions.
In a bowl, mix cooked quinoa, lemon zest, lemon juice, chopped parsley, and minced garlic.
Serve the baked cod on a bed of lemon and herb quinoa.
Nutritional Value:
High in omega-3 fatty acids, protein, and antioxidants.
Low in saturated fats.
Serving:
Serves 4
Cooking Time:
25 minutes
6. Vegetarian Lentil Soup
Ingredients:

1 cup dry green lentils, rinsed
1 onion, diced
2 carrots, diced
2 celery stalks, diced
3 cloves garlic, minced
1 can (14 oz) diced tomatoes
6 cups vegetable broth
1 teaspoon ground cumin
1 teaspoon smoked paprika
Salt and pepper to taste
Fresh cilantro for garnish

Preparation:

In a large pot, sauté onion, carrots, celery, and garlic until softened.

Add lentils, diced tomatoes, vegetable broth, cumin, smoked paprika, salt, and pepper.

Bring to a boil, then reduce heat and simmer for 25-30 minutes or until lentils are tender.

Garnish with fresh cilantro before serving.

Nutritional Value:

High in fiber, plant-based protein, and essential nutrients. Low in saturated fats.

Serving:

Serves 6-8

Cooking Time:

40 minutes

7. Turkey and Vegetable Skewers with Quinoa
Ingredients:

1 lb lean ground turkey
1 red onion, cut into chunks
1 bell pepper (any color), cut into chunks
1 zucchini, sliced
1 cup cherry tomatoes
2 tablespoons olive oil
1 teaspoon dried rosemary
1 teaspoon smoked paprika
Salt and pepper to taste
1 cup cooked quinoa

Preparation:

Preheat the grill or grill pan.

In a bowl, mix ground turkey with dried rosemary, smoked paprika, salt, and pepper. Form into small meatballs.

Thread meatballs, red onion, bell pepper, zucchini, and cherry tomatoes onto skewers.

Brush skewers with olive oil and grill for 12-15 minutes, turning occasionally until turkey is cooked through and veggies are charred.

Serve over a bed of cooked quinoa.

Nutritional Value:

High in lean protein, fiber, and antioxidants.

Low in saturated fats.

Serving:

Serves 4

Cooking Time:

25 minutes

8. Spinach and Mushroom Stuffed Chicken Breast

Ingredients:

4 boneless, skinless chicken breasts

2 cups fresh spinach, chopped

1 cup mushrooms, finely chopped

1/2 cup feta cheese, crumbled

2 cloves garlic, minced

1 tablespoon olive oil

1 teaspoon dried thyme

Salt and pepper to taste

Preparation:

Preheat the oven to 375°F.

In a skillet, sauté mushrooms and garlic in olive oil until softened. Add chopped spinach and cook until wilted. Remove from heat.

Butterfly each chicken breast and stuff with the spinach and mushroom mixture. Sprinkle feta cheese on top.

Season each stuffed chicken breast with dried thyme, salt, and pepper.

Bake in the oven for 25-30 minutes or until the chicken is cooked through.

Nutritional Value:

High in protein, iron, and vitamins.

Provides a good balance of healthy fats.

Serving:

Serves 4

Cooking Time:

35 minutes

9. Vegetarian Chickpea and Spinach Curry

Ingredients:

2 cans (15 oz each) chickpeas, drained and rinsed

1 onion, finely chopped

2 tomatoes, diced

3 cups fresh spinach

1 can (14 oz) coconut milk

2 tablespoons olive oil

2 teaspoons curry powder

1 teaspoon turmeric

1 teaspoon cumin

Salt and pepper to taste

Cooked brown rice for serving

Preparation:

In a large pot, sauté chopped onion in olive oil until translucent.

Add curry powder, turmeric, and cumin. Stir well.

Add diced tomatoes and cook until they break down.

Pour in coconut milk and bring to a simmer.

Stir in chickpeas and cook for 10-15 minutes.

Add fresh spinach and cook until wilted.

Season with salt and pepper. Serve over cooked brown rice.

Nutritional Value:

Rich in plant-based protein, fiber, and antioxidants.

Provides a good source of iron.

Serving:

Serves 4-6

Cooking Time:

30 minutes

10. Mediterranean Turkey and Quinoa Stuffed Peppers

Ingredients:

4 bell peppers (any color), halved and seeds removed

1 lb lean ground turkey

1 cup cooked quinoa

1 cup cherry tomatoes, halved

1/2 cup Kalamata olives, chopped

1/2 cup feta cheese, crumbled

2 tablespoons olive oil

1 teaspoon dried oregano

Salt and pepper to taste

Preparation:

Preheat the oven to 375°F.

In a skillet, brown ground turkey in olive oil. Season with dried oregano, salt, and pepper.

In a large bowl, mix cooked quinoa, cherry tomatoes, olives, and feta cheese.

Fill each bell pepper half with the turkey mixture.

Bake for 25-30 minutes or until peppers are tender.

Garnish with additional feta and fresh oregano if desired.

Nutritional Value:

High in lean protein, fiber, and Mediterranean flavors.

Provides essential vitamins and minerals.

Serving:

Serves 4

Cooking Time:

40 minutes

STANDARD KITCHEN MEASUREMENTS AND THEIR EQUIVALENCE.

1. Teaspoon (tsp)
- Equal to 5 milliliters (ml)
- Typically employed for modest quantities of spices, extracts, or fluid elements like honey.

2. Tablespoon (tbsp)
- Equal to 15 milliliters (ml) or 3 teaspoons
- Utilized for more substantial amounts of ingredients such as condiments, oils, or sauces.

3. Cup
- Equal to 240 milliliters (ml)
- A conventional measure for both dry and liquid components like flour, sugar, or milk.

4. Fluid Ounce (Fl oz)
- Equal to 30 milliliters (ml)
- Utilized for gauging liquids such as water, juice, or milk.

5. Pint
- Equal to 16 fluid ounces or roughly 473 milliliters
- Commonly used for quantifying liquids in larger volumes.

6. Quart
- Equal to 32 fluid ounces or approximately 946 milliliters
- Frequently employed for more substantial liquid volumes in cooking or baking.

7. Gallon
- Equal to 128 fluid ounces or about 3,785 milliliters
- A larger unit applied for measuring bulk liquid volumes.

8. Ounce (oz)
- Equal to approximately 28.35 grams
- Utilized for measuring both dry and liquid ingredients, particularly in smaller amounts.

9. Pound (lb.)
- Equal to 16 ounces or roughly 453.592 grams
- Typically used for measuring larger quantities of ingredients like flour, sugar, or meat.

10. Gram (g)
- A metric unit of weight, frequently used for precision in measurements.
- Approximately 28.35 grams make up one ounce.

11. Milligram (mg)
- A smaller unit of weight, especially beneficial for measuring supplements or specific additives.
- One gram is equivalent to 1,000 milligrams.

CONCLUSION

In conclusion, this MIND Disease Diet Cookbook for seniors over 60 is not just a compilation of recipes; it's a journey towards nurturing your brain health and overall well-being. Through these carefully crafted recipes, we've aimed to make adopting the MIND diet a delightful and flavorful experience.

As you age, the importance of maintaining cognitive function becomes increasingly evident. The MIND diet, rich in brain-boosting nutrients, offers a proactive approach to promote mental acuity and guard against neurodegenerative diseases. The carefully curated recipes in this cookbook are not just nourishing for the body but also a celebration of the joy that mindful and nutritious eating can bring to our lives.

The simplicity of these recipes is intentional, acknowledging the potential challenges that cooking may present in later years. We believe that every meal is an opportunity to show love and care to oneself, and this cookbook serves as a guide to achieving just that.

So, dear reader, as you embark on this culinary adventure, remember that adopting and adapting to the MIND diet is a gift to your future self. It's a commitment to a healthier, sharper, and more vibrant you. Embrace the flavors, savor the moments, and relish in the knowledge that every bite is a step towards a brighter tomorrow.

In the words of the ancient philosopher, Seneca, "It's not that we have a short time to live, but that we waste much of it." Embrace this cookbook as a tool to make the most of your time, nourishing both body and mind.

As you explore the recipes and incorporate them into your lifestyle, we invite you to share your experience. Your journey matters, and your feedback is invaluable. Don't forget to leave a review on Amazon—a token of gratitude that fuels our commitment to enhancing the lives of seniors through mindful nutrition.

Thank you for choosing this cookbook. Here's to your health, happiness, and the joy of savoring every moment.

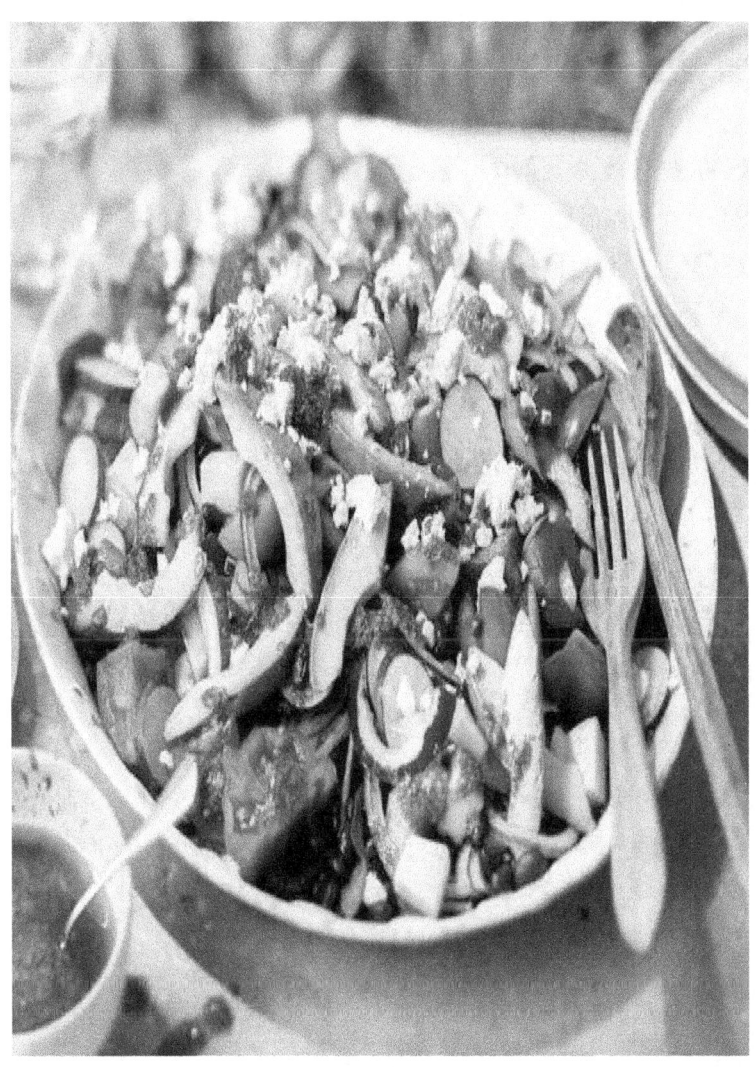

THANK YOU!!!

IF YOU FIND THIS BOOK TO BE INFORMATIVE, INSPIRING, OR SIMPLY ENJOYABLE, I WOULD BE IMMENSELY GRATEFUL IF YOU COULD SHARE YOUR THOUGHTS WITH OTHERS. YOUR HONEST REVIEW CAN MAKE A DIFFERENCE IN HELPING MORE INDIVIDUALS DISCOVER THE BENEFITS OF A NOURISHING AND MINDFUL APPROACH TO EATING. PLEASE CONSIDER LEAVING A REVIEW ON AMAZON AND SHARE YOUR EXPERIENCE.

THANK YOU ONCE AGAIN FOR CHOOSING THIS BOOK AS A COMPANION ON YOUR PATH TO A HEALTHIER, HAPPIER YOU.

7 WEEKS DIET MEAL PLANNER

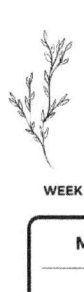
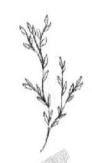

Daily Meal Planner

WEEK :   MONTH :   YEAR :

MONDAY	TUESDAY	WEDNESDAY

THURSDAY	FRIDAY	WEEKEND

NOTES

Daily Meal Planner

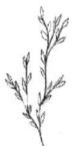 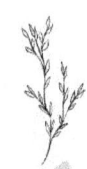

WEEK :   **MONTH :**   **YEAR :**

MONDAY	TUESDAY	WEDNESDAY

THURSDAY	FRIDAY	WEEKEND

NOTES

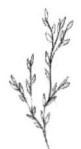

Daily Meal Planner

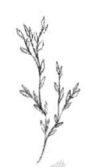

WEEK: MONTH: YEAR:

MONDAY	TUESDAY	WEDNESDAY

THURSDAY	FRIDAY	WEEKEND

NOTES

Daily Meal
Planner

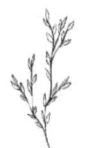
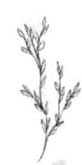

WEEK :   **MONTH :**   **YEAR :**

MONDAY	TUESDAY	WEDNESDAY

THURSDAY	FRIDAY	WEEKEND

NOTES

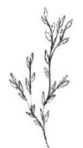

Daily Meal Planner

WEEK :   **MONTH :**   **YEAR :**

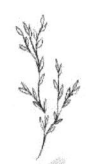

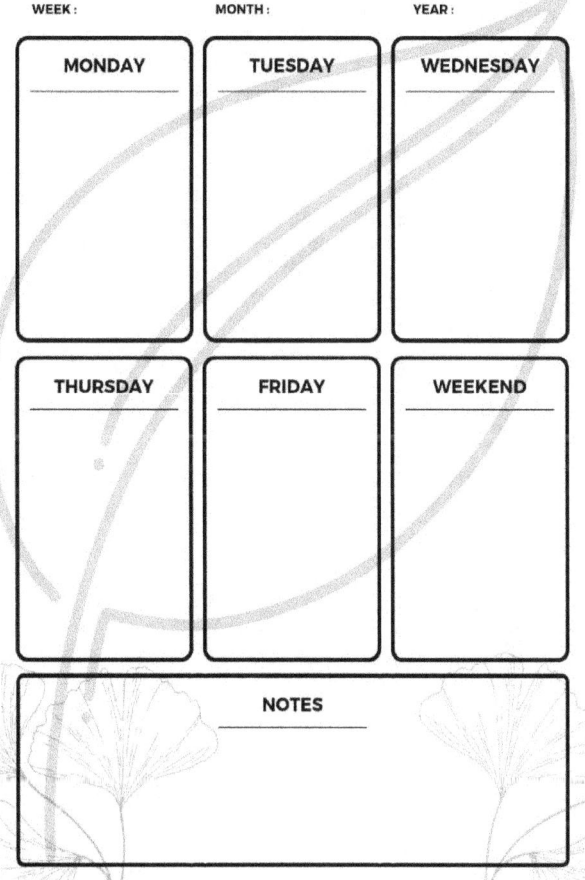

MONDAY

TUESDAY

WEDNESDAY

THURSDAY

FRIDAY

WEEKEND

NOTES

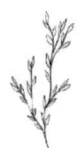 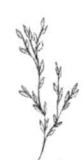

Daily Meal Planner

WEEK :   MONTH :   YEAR :

MONDAY	TUESDAY	WEDNESDAY

THURSDAY	FRIDAY	WEEKEND

NOTES

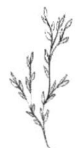

Daily Meal Planner

WEEK :   **MONTH :**   **YEAR :**

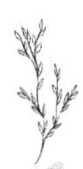

MONDAY	TUESDAY	WEDNESDAY

THURSDAY	FRIDAY	WEEKEND

NOTES